BIODYNAMICS OF OSTEOPATHY

Phase Six

Second Edition

James Jealous D.O.

For more information about Dr. Jealous please visit:
https://BiodynamicsOfOsteopathy.com

BIODYNAMICS OF OSTEOPATHY   Phase Six

Hardback ISBN: 979-8-2955-3929-9
eBook ISBN: 979-8-2955-5647-0

Second Edition 2025

James Jealous D.O. (1943–2021) practiced as an osteopathic physician, teacher and writer for many years. His life's work was to found and develop the specific methodology of Biodynamics of Osteopathy, following the lineage of Dr. A.T. Still and Dr. W.G. Sutherland.

This is one of a series of Biodynamics of Osteopathy books. They grew organically from sets of handouts written by Dr. Jealous and given to students during courses taught by him and his teachers. After many years he collected the handouts together and created individual course manuals, which he added to and rewrote many times. After several more years they evolved further into books.

TABLE OF CONTENTS

OSTEOPATHY IS SERVICE

We use our hands …

To treat the Whole patient

To listen to the indwelling movements of Life

To treat all levels of illness

To assist in building the patient's functional reserve

To support homeostasis and trophicity by balancing the activity of the autonomic nervous system

To explore "laws not framed by human hands" (Dr. Still and Dr. Sutherland)

To cooperate and communicate with the Laws of Nature (Dr. Wales)

"To find the Health" (Dr. Still)

To get to the treatment plan

To get to the diagnosis

To help establish a point of Rest or Neutral around which the Whole can come to balance

To find Cause

We believe ...

We have an innate capacity to heal
The patient functions as a whole
The autonomic nervous system plays a major role in disease and healing
Structure and function are one form of activity
The Divine is indwelling
Life moves beyond death
There is a Constant Movement toward Normal
We are here to Serve Humanity

Normal is ...

"A sense of peace and harmony" (Dr. Sutherland)
Ease of motion, without tension
A capacity for Neutral
A sense of Wholeness to Life
The capacity for adaptation, change without compensation.

"Skill is proportionate to one's understanding of normal" (Dr. Still)

THE MOVEMENT FROM PHASE ONE TO PHASE SIX

In **Phase One**, we began therapeutics that involved *involuntary motion in the lesion field*; we called this movement *motion present* and realized that this motion is an aspect of the Health ... the challenge we faced with this realization was that it became necessary to give a treatment without any barrier or leading the treatment tempo. The Direction of Ease we followed in the lesion led to neutral, where one could see tissue transmuted into fluid.

Phase Two focused on the fluid body (Zone B) and its dynamics at a rate of two to three cycles per minute. The fluid body has an infrastructure of protoplasm, which makes its study different than the study of water. Protoplasm is "the first moldable substance that can hold an image." We studied the neutral at this rate, and level two stillness, which created a treatment called automatic shifting.

The treatment was very detailed and diagnostic, as well as educational for the observer, who retained a relationship with the stillness throughout the process, so as not to inhibit the potential for transmutation. We discussed the role of neutral in ourselves and in our patients as a precursor to receiving the potency of primary respiration at deeper levels. At the end of the course, the Long-Tide was becoming apparent.

Phase Three focused on the fluid body at a rate of one hundred seconds per cycle (Long-Tide) and the indwelling presence of a therapeutic force in the lesion field. We noted that the therapeutic force can guide our attention.

Phase Four followed the truth of the midline. The Tide brought us to a deeper understanding of being centered by the Tide as Dr. Becker wrote about in the 1965 Sutherland Memorial Lecture. This is a major change for most of us because our intention is replaced by the intention of the Tide ... this echoes through our lives in many ways and creates a spiritual path that leads onward toward the cause behind the charity of the Tide.

Phase Five was centered around the head and neck. We explored the fluid field segments that we have appreciated through our research in Biodynamics ... we learned about not giving direction to our observations of the fluid fields. We worked with the seams as the functional primordial of the fluid fields. We saw the seams blend into a more primordial state of Dynamic Stillness (empty head full of luminous darkness) then, as we waited, spontaneous ignition occurred. The middle face fluid field was explored. The wholeness of fluid dynamics and the Fluid Body was stressed.

Phase Six is a continuation of our journey into the love and wholeness that generates life and delivers therapeutic forces that transmute lesions, once the neutral is expressed. We will continue to work with the Dynamic Stillness and the developmental fulcrum in the head. We will also explore the extremities. Phase Six is a mixture of activities centered around the outside presence of primary respiration as something that is a non-biological force that has a persona. We will also look at seams again and then move on to the extremities, first in the embryological terms, then as Sutherland taught them in his work called Power Points ... Phase Six is a time to build your understanding of the Tide and refine your skills. Phase Seven is only about the Health.

THE PAUSE ... BEFORE THE SONG

Phases Five and Six are designed to allow your perception to become dependent upon the Tide.

In Phase Four we began noticing that the Tide can "center us" in a much deeper manner than when we use our own will to center ourselves. This, of course, is one of the functions of midline dynamics ... to center us. We then entered Phase Five, where we continued to allow this "centering and healing" to occur while we remained relatively neutral. Phase Six continues this attention to a dependency on the Tide. While we are transitioning our perception to this dependency, we will continue to explore areas of interest. In Phase Six, we will study the extremities as Sutherland approached them with his study group. This information has never been taught outside of his private group except in these courses. The information came from Ruby Day, D.O., who was with Sutherland from 1935 to the end of his life.

Becoming neutral and waiting to be centered by the Tide is not as easy as it sounds. It requires patience. We have mental and emotional habits that reflexively jump out when stimulated. We do not reject or feel disgust toward our habits ... this only increases the lesions. We need to remain neutral in the face of adversity. We have therefore not changed the perceptual studies in Phases Four through Six, in order to give ourselves the necessary time to change under the influence of the Tide.

As we come under the sweet presence of the Tide, we will begin to leave the zones behind and enter a more universal space. Space is a real place. It is the beginning of Life. We saw this in the seams of the face when they coalesced into an "empty head" ... we noted that ignition was spontaneous when this level of neutral was expressed in the patient.

Our principle of rebalancing also takes on another form as we see the world through the eyes of the Tide. We have become aware that Zone B is a child of a great maternal ocean and that the connection is sustained throughout life. The "flow" between the mother and child is a central river that we call the midline.

All these principles come from studying Dr. Sutherland's work and the words of Dr. Becker in his 1965 Sutherland Memorial Lecture, "Be Still and Know." The quote "Be still and know that I am God" is from Psalm 46. It is about being centered and willed by God, not oneself. This is a deeply elevated state of being. It reflects God communicating and centering us ... it comes out of the blue ... we do not add anything of our own to this event.

We must be in love and become neutral, then the stage is set for higher intervention.

"We must learn to reawaken and keep ourselves awake ... by an infinite expectation of the dawn, which does not forsake us in our soundest sleep.
(Thoreau)

Rebalance through the relationship of the Fluid Body to the Dynamic Stillness in the sea around and through us.

PHASE SIX COMMENTS

The unfolding of our form and function is a Mystery. We can, however, see certain relationships. One that is remarkable is the relationship of the presence of primary respiration in the sea around us to the individual fulcrums of specific functions.

The presence in the sea is different than the Long-Tide or the Dynamic Stillness. In Phases Three, Four, and Five, we studied the Long-Tide and the dynamic stillness as therapeutic forces. Now we come to a new set of principles that reveal an essential relationship in healing. This relationship is about the presence, the sense of living wisdom and love that creates our form and function. At first it appears to be outside of us, and the fulcrum inside, but the spatial sense of this will change as we work with it. It does not move from one place to another like the Long-Tide, and it has an intelligence that works now.

Our health is borne from the Sea Around Us. We could say that each function and form have a seed from the sea, and as it unfolds we see growth and developmental locally, as well as in the whole. We will see this in our work in Phase Six.

The fulcrum of origin is larger and deeper than the anatomy it gives birth to. We will see that using anatomy as a landmark for locating the seed will not reveal the relationship we are interested in.

The neutrals that proceed from this relationship are associated with ignition.

By now you should be familiar with the following:

- Fire in the bones
- Slow ignition (Long-Tide)
- The "bird"
- The "wire"

Primary respiration and thoracic respiration co-emerge as one breathing in the embryo. Healthy children retain this. In adults these are separate. As we heal, they return to their original fulcrum.

As a practical, synchronize the following:

- Thoracic respiration and its fulcrum
- Primary respiration, and its fulcrum
- The stillness upon which they rest ... the original fulcrum
- Emergence of one breath, the "embryonic breath"

Our consciousness is a gift. We do not own it. If we control it, we lose our wholeness. We become isolated from the love and sweetness of creation. Since Phase Four, we have stressed how important this is.

REBALANCING, PHASE ONE TO PHASE FOUR

The Fulcrum as a Doorway

- Fulcrums are interlinked by the Health precognitively.
- A breezeway of Ease, or gently impassible.
- An extension of the Direction of Ease in the lesion field.
- The lesion field is alive, using energy all day.

Cause

Find the cause of symptoms, or signs of dysfunction:

- Shingles is not a cause.
- Ulcers are not a cause.
- Cancer is not a cause.
- Hypertension is not a cause.

FINDING CAUSE ...

Osteopathy was a new science of healing. It did not begin as a subspecialty of Allopathic medicine. This new science had a unique and effective philosophy, which could be applied by those with skilled senses.

The premise of Osteopathy is that we have the means to heal ourselves. The medicine is, and can be, manufactured by our own inner resources. Our work with primary respiration has proven this premise time and time again.

The principle we will address here is "finding cause."

In Osteopathy, the cause is much deeper than the symptoms. In Allopathic applications, the symptoms are the cause that one addresses for the cure. However superficial this may appear to any reasonable mind, the fact is that this is the general application of "cure."

All schools of healing common in today's Western culture have adopted this mindset that has seeped into all categories of higher education ... including Osteopathy. I can appreciate that superficial symptoms are important to the patient, and I am not proposing that we should not aim to remove the cause of the symptoms ... but what is the cause?

How deep can one go to find cause without producing stress in the whole patient?

Primary respiration can communicate this to us and is an invaluable tool in helping us find cause.

We will focus on tracking the cause.

Finding the cause through history taking is another topic that will be addressed later.

CAUSE

Our profession is grounded in a unique philosophy and methodology.

We do not believe that the disease is a cause, but a symptom of a deeper disproportion.

We have all heard these words, but most Osteopaths remain unable to see the signs and symptoms presented by the patient as part of a deeper cause that must be addressed.

If someone complains of a frozen shoulder, then it is treated as the cause of his or her dysfunction, when in fact we have done nothing to find out why the patient is ill other than be led around by a history that embraces the superficial. The patient says, "I overused my arm doing such and such." The reductionist in us is happy and feels like a real doctor making such superficial connections. This is not Osteopathy.

When I was in Kirksville in 1965, it was impressed upon me over and over again that the symptoms were not the illness. Anyone can make simple conclusions. Anyone can find disease and label it.

Still saw into the human organism much more deeply. What was he pointing at and how do we begin to explore this principle of finding cause?

Cause in a reductionist framework is an isolated force event. Effect is what comes from the cause. Things do not arise just from local causes and current events. The whole life of the patient is the stage upon which insult occurs.

Any lesion that has not been transmuted remains in us. These lesions are not asleep; inert, they grow every day in the darkness of an unconscious world.

Lesions are dynamic; they are alive. They use up tremendous energy.

Lesions continue to grow until the Tide brings them into view at a moment when the whole heals.

The power and the timing for the conversion of a lesion comes from the Tide. This is a principle of healing. It cannot be forced into resolution.

The power to integrate comes from the functional reserve the patient has in the whole. Functional reserve is a day-to-day repository of life forces, but there could be a lesion draining the reserve as fast as it fills ... this most often leads to addiction and dependency on others for energy and identity. Caution: being a psychologist is of no help here ... it may make the lesion deepen.

Now we will begin to find cause. The trail we follow is dictated by the health, which will not let us tread where our logic wants to go. The Tide will protect the patient from self-observation while it transmutes the lesion field.

THE FULCRUM

Practical

Chief complaint ... anything, not just structural.

Find the lesion field ... and the boundaries.

Find the force vectors and follow them to the fulcrum.

Pass through the fulcrum as if it is a doorway.

It will bring you to a new area, a new lesion field.

Go to the area.

Find the boundaries and the force vectors.

Find the fulcrum.

Can you easily pass through the doorway or does the Tide stop your progress?

Continue from place to place until the Tide will not let you through the doorway.

Then treat the patient here, not at the area of the chief complaint.

Recheck in five to six weeks.

Neutral is idling; it is not flaccid.

It is alive and ready.

It is a finely tuned state of reserve that is met by an outside influence, which shifts it into action. It has no will of its own.

****Thanks to the research by Karen Gadja, D.O., we know that the idea of neutral, or idling, appears in Fryette's work as early as 1915.*

MEDITATION

We will watch some of the gifts we are blessed with as a result of being created.

The Observer

We are given the capacity to observe creation as it occurs.

Generally, the observer is fixed ... unable to be freely shifted by life and the Tide as it unfolds. There are very great implications to this freedom: a neutral heart, inner peace, and love.

Consider the reality that "you are not your observer."

You do not need to observe. It is done for you, like your breathing. Please watch for the automatic shifting of the observer as a movement of the Tide rather than habit during this time of meditation. The intrinsic motion of a free observer is to be centered and stilled by the breath of life, then everything is one motion.

Awareness can unfold like an embryo

The Breathing of Thoracic Respiration

Here is something that reveals the nature of our dullness.

We are to be breathed, in/out, in/out, with an intimacy that would shock most people. Inside of you is the great movement of life ... not a machine, but a moment-to-moment awakening of existence. Death/birth repeating a drama that allows growth and healing by ending the past and allowing the future only seconds to exist before it dies.

Just watch the coming and going ... and see where this leads

The Sea Around Us

We are watching this Sea and the breathing of the Long-Tide. It is an ocean. In the shoreline of the horizon the fluid breathes. It passes through the material world as if it was transparent. The awareness of this is aboriginal. It is normal to feel it. It is spoken of as a Divine mother in many traditions. The sensation of this presence is very intimate and carries with it a sense of nurture and shelter. It transforms isolation. One's response is restful. Then the ocean expands.

The Stillness of Zone C

There is a stillness always present in Zone C, which is our place of reverence for the Divine. It can be felt in the heart and indwelling sanctuary.

Automatic Shifting

As we watch the above individual activities, the one that is in the foreground will automatically shift. As we said above, let the focus of your attention be free; do not move it around; it will move by itself toward healing and wholeness. This is important to see.

Rest

What do you do?

Nothing but rest and watch ... let the Tide have the fulcrum of intention, then you will just be resting (neutral) and in good company.

Footnotes

Our breathing is usually an effect of our inner state of mind: thoughts, fears, images; our mental engine is unstable, flitting about, identifying every movement as "me."

When we bring our attention to the above landscapes and let the awareness unfold by its own intelligence, it will follow one landscape then another, automatically shifting while you just hold your intention to be restful and neutral.

The mind, at a higher level, unites the four landscapes into one. Without our knowing it, this other-mind is aware of the fulcrum around which all four coexist as one. This other-mind will carry you to a deeper resting place, a central stillness upon which all breath becomes one and from which we are born. It is the health at work in us, guiding the meditation. Sometimes it gets warm.

As we are guided, distractions will enter. Do not resist distractions. Remain neutral. Let the Tide move the meditation. As the meditation moves along, the rates change in both primary and thoracic respiration, things slow down, the sympathetic tone in us diminishes ... ease occurs ... then the breathing pauses by itself. We may be breathless for a moment, but something is feeding us, uniting us.

RESUSCITATION OF THE PATIENT

There are a variety of resuscitation methods that we have explored throughout the Phases. The one we engage with today is for a particular type of patient: the patient who has felt their own health, identified their self as self, and felt a presence that centered them (healed).

The moment when one is touched by the presence of the Tide, one becomes transparent to the beauty of love that places each of us at the center of eternity. In these moments one communicates with the divine in some secret room that the clinician cannot see.

It became common in my practice as a general practitioner to have patients call for an appointment and, as they came into the treatment room, to say, "I am not sick but I miss the feeling of that presence. I miss God. Can you help me find that relationship again?"

The request took many forms ... I never questioned their validity.

In each case, I could remember clearly the moment when that particular person, while in treatment, connected to the beauty and persona of the incarnate health in themselves as a deep veil fell over them, hiding the content of events from my eyes.

Then came ...

> The sensation in the "linking up" with the divine.
>
> A sense of activity in the third ventricle that extended to an outside presence that lay in the perfect heart ...
>
> A sense of the patient awakened in the stars, at home.
>
> The long lever, reaching to a fulcrum, known as mystery to our minds but known as beloved to our hearts.
>
> In the presence of that presence comes a wholeness, a healing ...

Something that supersedes any personal suffering that is in isolation from the warmth of that presence.

The sensation of which eclipses all of our pain from any cause.

The myriad of times I have seen this, there always seems to be a sense of the extension of the patient's mind (third ventricle) toward the outside, toward a presence that lives for us in the stars.

Always, as this happened, I had the thought, "they are healed." And usually their clinical symptoms cleared ...

Remember, these were people I knew for many years ... I do not want you to think that this point was reached miraculously, in one treatment; it was through many treatments and hard work by the patient to heal using all parameters of mental attitude, diet, exercise, and personal self- discovery, and, infrequently, medication for brief periods of time.

When patients returned, I was surprised, having thought that once they found the health, they would not need my services again.

But old habits would creep in ... the psyche would engage "cause and effect" as reality and settle back into a duality within itself.

Even though the patients' health had not declined, their sense of normal was the awareness of a living divinity. Without that sense, they felt out of balance and pursued resolution through treatment.

All my knowledge of these things I learned from my patients and their experience ... I never indicated to any of them that these things could happen ... I followed them and the Tide as my teacher ... this was not a belief system that I went into practice with.

One of the interesting perceptual shifts in Sutherland was when he felt the divine presence and began to refer to the Tide as "Dad" ... to me this speaks of an innocent sense of being loved and guided by a higher mind, the one Dr. Still refers to so often.

When a patient requested this kind of "tune-up" ... I had no idea of what to do ... when I checked them, there were no outstanding lesions. Maybe the vitality was a little low. Maybe the ignition was a little down … but really nothing to be called a lesion. There was a certain level of wholeness.

As I matured in practice, I could see a pattern in the style of treatment the Tide created to bring the patient's perception in line with awareness of the divine.

THE OUTSIDE PRESENCE

Practical

Let the patient pursue neutral on their own. Usually I tell them, "Go lie down and go to neutral ... I will be along." ... They do.

When I arrive several minutes later, they are transmuting toward neutral.

They will transmute through a two-to-three-cycle-per-minute level neutral to a neutral on the Long-Tide ... this happens slowly and easily over a few minutes.

As they plateau at the Long-Tide neutral, they then begin to stall in their momentum toward a deeper neutral within the dynamic stillness. If they could go all the way, they would not need treatment.

Our task, therefore, is to wait at the neutral for the dynamic stillness, for them to come to that place, not follow them ... we wait in this place where they will arrive later.

Our waiting at this neutral is the treatment. Our mind is centered outside in the outside presence of the sea around us ... do not sense anything inside even though you see the dynamic stillness neutral place as inside the patient.

Our perceptual fulcrum is outside, not in the patient.

The outside presence is not the Long-Tide or the dynamic stillness, but a mind that sees through everything ... as the Buddhists say, "the hand of compassion." As the Christians say, "God's love."

As the patient comes into the Dynamic Stillness neutral, they slowly become formless, and as they do you will feel a moment when the mind of the patient hooks into a faraway place ... and then we see nothing ...

the meeting is sacred, hidden from us.

Once they hook up, our hands are quietly removed as the healing occurs in a manner not visible to us.

Later, perhaps twenty minutes … the patient stirs.

The discipline in Phase Six is to hold your attention outside with the presence of the deity that centers us.

SEAMS

At the end of Phase Five we looked at the middle face seam. This is a very important seam in many ways, including for understanding the sinuses and the upper dental arch.

Seams are everywhere.

They appear in protoplasm, as spaces opening in formlessness.

The seams provide the geometric basis of form.

FURTHER COMMENTS ON SEAMS

The essential feature of a seam is space, not the space between anatomical landmarks.

Space is a specific state of life into which the invisible matrix of the health begins orderly growth.

Space is bigger than the function it creates.

Therapeutic forces recognize seams as they frequently disappear into a seam before the seams merge into pure space.

The therapeutic forces one engages in a seam vary from the Long-Tide and the dynamic stillness to the liquid light of the health.

Space is a rich dark substance. Still said, "Life is that substance which fills all the spaces of the universe."

Dr. Schooley mentions these principles in his article "Fulcrums." See the 1953 OCA Journal.

There are three types of seams recognized in clinical practice:

The anatomical seam is recognizable as a location, such as the seam between the upper and middle face, which can be identified by following a series of landmarks. If one begins anteriorly at nasion, one can palpate a seam that goes laterally through the orbit and the eyes into the zygomatic-frontal suture. The seam then passes through the disc of the temporomandibular joint (TMJ) in the temporal fossa and along the squamous petrous junction as it passes gently above the outer ear. From there it continues above mastoid process, through asterion and on into the transverse sinus. There are some genetic variants, but the pattern is quite clear when palpated on a living person. The underlying intracranial structures are also on this seam.

Another seam is called the functional seam. This is in the fluid field (Zone B). It is the place from which the seam actually functions in a particular patient. It is most often a considerable distance (inches) from the anatomical seam. Finding the functional seam is how we make decisions on where to treat and assess the progress of a series of treatments.

The third type of seam we call the seam of the health. This seam is perfect. It has no anatomical position where you can sense its presence. It is where it is. Because we are so addicted to anatomy as a reference point, we often find this seam displaced... it is not displaced, the anatomy is displaced. Becoming aligned with this healthy seam and its truth changes many things.

Discernment of these seams requires practice. At least fifty cases are needed to get the "feel" of these things. One must apply new principles, but most important is the death of the old habits and convergent thinking.

Perception in this realm depends on mental neutrality and being "centered by the Tide." This is not easy and is a challenging step. It could take many years to attain a naturally neutral awareness. One must desire the change for concrete reasons or nothing can happen. Our brains can only repattern if we are neutral. This allows neuroplasticity to express its dynamics.

THE TREATMENT OF INTRAORAL LESIONS WITHOUT DIRECT ACTION

The history of cranial technique has followed two rivers, one direct and one indirect.

In Phase Three we discussed the anterior dural girdle fluid field. As you may remember, the halo around the cranial end of the midline of the embryonic plate (angiogenetic cluster) descends as a fluid wave to create the diaphragm, heart, lungs, foregut, liver, and other functions at predetermined locations, established by the movement of the whole embryo.

The same fluid field creates all functions from the bregma to the xiphoid, including the fluid field segments we explored in Phase Five.

If you can imagine an egg-shaped area from the top of the head to just below the diaphragm, empty of anatomy, then you can appreciate a unit of function being expressed from the anterior dural girdle fluid field.

The Tide continues to teach us new formats and designs that dissolve our anatomical limits into a world untapped by science—a world that A. T. Still clearly saw, as did his colleague W. G. Sutherland.

The map is not in any book ... it is in your patients ... watch ... if you see a repetitious therapeutic force or pathway, remember it. Write it down.

It does little good to learn embryology and superimpose it on the patient or the primary respiration ... all that comes from imposition is bad habits and limitations for us all ... just watch nature ... and remember ... the story will gain in memory from the source itself ... really.

The fluid will follow a matrix that is invisible, except for the wake left in the fluid field as it passes under the power of the potency of transmutation.

Listen to your imagination, as Sutherland has told us to ...

Imagination is a form of knowing that exceeds the intellect. It is a higher function.

Trust what you see and your imagination will carry you into a conversation with the Tide ... and a conversion of your senses.

Who came to this truth but great thinkers like Socrates and Plato, who were and are respected as "exceptional" ... meet the challenge in yourself of using a higher faculty ... see beyond the rigidity of books and expert opinions ... become free, test the value of trust ... then decide what is the true nature of the imagination. An image is created in our mind by the motion of the therapeutic forces ... like skywriting by an airplane ... we do not make the writing; the natural world inscribes it for us...the image is formed by the real use of our senses. A real form of knowing.

Study and you will see that your fear of being fooled by your imagination is what has fooled you into thinking that way.

Practical

The lower middle face and the anterior dural girdle are two intersecting areas (see schematic below).

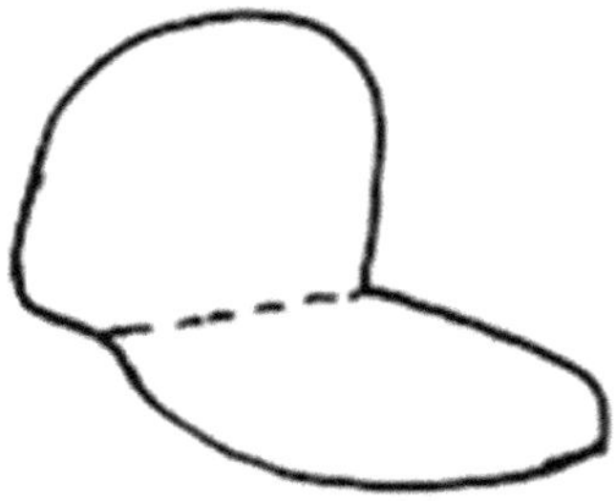

The anatomical interface occurs at the junction of the pterygoid processes of the sphenoid and the immaculate palatine bones ... this area is worth studying with the individual bones in hand, because it is one of the most beautiful articulations in the body. The palatine is inspiring to study, it being so fragile and so woven into so many functions. As you sense this interface, feel for distortion of form and function ... it will be clear if any anatomical stress is present.

As you know, there are congenital cleft palates and dental lesions, and children often have things like pencils in their mouths that get jammed forcefully into the soft and hard palates, leaving considerable disruption. This area also gets distorted whenever there is any trauma to the vault ... see Phase Three, the periosteal sac.

The functional activity involves the fluid fields locally and how they connect to the egg-shaped space described above and ultimately to the whole of Zone B (the fluid body). As you sense for the breathing of primary respiration in this fluid field, you may feel aberrant fluid fluctuations and/or a displacement between the anatomy (Zone A) and the fluid field (Zone B) ... sometimes the fulcrums for each are very far apart.

The biodynamic relationship to this area and the whole is sensed through the relationship between the central fulcrum and the outside presence of primary respiration that created it ... this is where the word Biodynamics originates in our work.

We will use this knowledge as we treat, centering our attention on the emptiness in the head and its egg-shaped fulcrum at the center. We are not engaging the fluid field or the anatomy, just the biodynamic level of the seed and the ocean that it comes from.

Once you have established an awareness of the egg and the outside presence, discipline your mind to stay only with the outside presence ... you will notice internal processes ... do not hook into them.

You will see activity from the diaphragm to the top of the head, demonstrating that the lesion is not local but is in the bigger space through which the form and function arose and continue to unfold as a wholeness.

In the biomechanical model, your action is direct and local. The thinking is that nerves are impinged upon by bones. If you had a child with dysphagia or poor speech development, you would go to the jugular foramen to release nerve pressure ... in the biodynamic model we go to a more fundamental cause and let the whole rebalance ... the motive for my mentioning this is that when treating upper dental arch problems in children, the release that unlocks the dental arch is often way down in the diaphragm fluid field. The release is a wave, not a tissue force vector.

As you work with this easy principle, many cases will be helped with immediacy and not long multiple treatments. The speed of recovery is greater, and that in itself speaks of a more refined process.

Be aware that I am giving you a handhold to begin with, but as your communication and trust grow, your hands will work differently, as the Tide will direct their attitude in any given patient.

FURTHER COMMENTS ON INTRAORAL STRAINS

This section is on a method of working that replaces intraoral technique. It involves understanding the relationship between the outside presence of primary respiration and the central fulcrum for the whole head. In Phase Five we observed the head void of anatomy and fluid fields, just a dark empty head. At the center of this emptiness was an egg-shaped space, a tone less dark than its surroundings. A fulcrum the size of a quail's egg. This fulcrum is central to this whole region and the thorax. It is like a seed from which unfolding takes place.

With our hands we will contact the upper dental arch and the region on the anterior dural girdle juxtaposed to the coronal suture. This particular hand position is just a doorway to a larger reality. This is an anatomical beginning that we will mentally disassociate from during treatment. The fluid fields are much greater than local anatomical landmarks. For example, the anterior dural girdle is not a tissue but rather a fluid field that extends its influence from the vault to below the diaphragm ... so ... during treatment we must be aware of a large area.

The functional interface between the upper dental arch and the anterior dural girdle is the place where the palatines and the pterygoid plates grow and develop. Remember, the sphenoid grows out of the anterior dural fluid field, as do the palatines ... think about this sincerely. This interface between the two arches is an important area to study in detail. Understanding this, and the conceptual fulcrum for the whole movement of the fluid field, opens a doorway to a functional and biodynamic treatment for a large area, including those previously corrected using intraoral techniques as described by Sutherland and Magoun.

Some clinical situations where this approach can help:

- Sinus problems
- Adenoid and tonsillar problems
- Hiatal hernia
- Hiccups
- Regurgitation

Treatment:

Align with the anatomy to sense any overt structural deformity.

Then sense the functional aspect of the space, the arches and the central fulcrum in the empty head … then become aware of the outside presence of Primary Respiration, and apply more of your attention outside, to this presence, and wait … but this time watch the treatment activity in the fluid fields so you can see the fluid dynamics at work and understand the fluid mind. Sense the whole fluid body from bregma to xiphoid.

The treatment often directs itself away from the area of pathology and alerts us to the "cause behind the cause" … for example, a child with large adenoids may demonstrate, during treatment, a release on the vertical height of the fluid field from xiphoid to bregma, informing us that the problem involves a larger area than the symptoms suggest … this is extremely helpful.

THE OUTSIDE PRESENCE OF PRIMARY RESPIRATION AND THE INNER FULCRUM OF UNFOLDING FOR THE HEAD AND THORAX

We have reviewed the different forms of respiration inherent to different levels of activity in both thoracic and primary respiration. We also recognized that these two forms of breathing co-emerge as one and later are broken into levels by the separation of the individual from the health. We can pursue an understanding of this one embryonic breath by personal observation in ourselves (contemplation). More on this in Phases Seven and Eight.

During the practical, we explored a principle of treatment. We brought the fulcrum in an "empty" head into our awareness and simultaneously were aware of the presence in the sea around us. No effort was made to connect them, as they are already one.

Usually, the therapeutic effects of this type of treatment are a neutral on the Long-Tide before treatment that transmutes to a neutral in the dynamic stillness, and a sense of formlessness in the patient. Soon after, there is a sense of the "third eye" (third ventricle) reconnecting with the presence of primary respiration in the stars (this is the moment when the patient returns to a perceptual awareness related to an intimate sense of love and safety ... this is why they came), and sometimes there is luminosity.

The end point is a mystery, as the patient is now in a secret chamber with the Tide. We can know when to take our hands off the patient because the presence will tell us, either directly or by shifting our consciousness.

There is no indication from the patient of when we are done.

The type of patient who responds to this is healthy. This is really a form of rebalancing, not resuscitation or treatment. This is the kind of patient who has personally felt the persona of the Tide and recognized its compassion.

Today we return to this principle of treatment as a replacement for intraoral technique. This time it will be a true treatment process, not a rebalancing; the patient is usually not equipped to have their third eye restored. The treatment will show the embryological fluid field relationships that validate the teaching of Blechschmidt and Sutherland.

This approach is appreciative of the relationship between the anterior dural girdle fluid field and the upper dental arch ... this is diagramed on the board. Please remember that the anterior girdle is a fluid field that is not restricted to the dural duplication of the sphenoparietal sinus.

Clinical settings in which this can be effective are sinusitis, enlarged adenoids, enlarged tonsils, palatine injuries, oropharyngeal somatic dysfunctions, hiccups, hiatal hernia, dysphagia, snoring (functional), and loss of vertical height in the fluid field from bregma to xiphoid ... it is used in adolescents a lot for acute upper respiratory problems, as the lymphatic drainage for the whole region is effected through fluid field dynamics and neutral (see WGS and his relationship with neutral and inflammatory resolution).

The treatment is arranged around the fulcrum at the center and the Outside Presence of Primary Respiration. The feel of this may be a little different than how it was before, because often patients are seen for acute intervention and their neutrals are weak. There may be more fluid in the awareness and less dynamic stillness. Often, we get some slow molding effects in the head and thorax as the Tide sorts out the wholeness of the lesion. For example, the area that releases could be the diaphragm fluid field even though the clinical symptoms may be in the tonsils. We will learn a lot about embryology as we watch the treatment reveal the facts of how the Health sees itself.

It's the not-yet in the now,

the taste of the fruit that does not-yet exist,

hanging the blossom on the bough."

–Laurens van der Post, Venture to the Interior

THE EXTREMITIES

We have learned a great deal from Sutherland's later work on the extremities. I will detail the history of that work later in our second practical on the extremities.

There are times, in practice, when we want to look at the whole extremity and its integrity. There is wholeness to a limb that includes both limbs as a unit of function.

This wholeness is vital to the repair of a damaged extremity and its resynchronization process, where the interplay of muscles, ligaments, and embracing membranes have a common fulcrum from which the wholeness can flow as the extremity moves. We have used Sutherland's work on Power Points, his work on fluid dynamics, and a knowledge of basic embryology to find a method that engages the whole extremity and not the parts.

Rebuilding an extremity is about its function, not its structure. Why? Because a muscle in an extremity does not arise from a notochord segment and migrate ... it arises from the local fluid in a specific location. For example, the brachioradialis muscle arises from the fluid in that location. The fluid shapes itself into the form of the muscle from whence it functions. The shape of the muscle IS its function.

No rigid structure is found unless the fluid field locks up and cannot express neutral.

The fluid field that forms all the muscles and connective tissue is one drop. Then it develops seams that we call facial planes, and shapes we call muscles, ligaments, et al. But ... but ... is the fluid centered around the midline of the extremity in a functional manner ... and ...

where is the fulcrum for the function of the whole extremity ... and ... where does this midline intersect with the notochord midline of the trunk ... from whence the limb was borne as a bud? All these things went into the creation of a limb ... are they correct in your patient?

Let's Think Osteopathy. If a damaged muscle needs to reform, rebuild, and resynchronize as a part of a myriad of symphonic activity, how is that accomplished in a healthy arm? Well, neutral is established in the whole, then automatic shifting until all functions (parts) have reoriented to the midline and its fulcrum. Then, at the central fulcrum, the two extremities become one, a single expression from a single fulcrum that buds in two directions from one seed ... one, not two, separate functions. There is only one arm and one leg ... these single images appear as two images ... but it is one image placed on two sides.

What about a patient who does not have these qualities at work in the extremity? Can we help these parts realign, resynchronize, repair, and transmute so that the fluid field is not stuck in the altered state and withering? Certainly.

The method must be precise.

Clinically, we see cases of crushed extremities. We see burn cases. We see growth delay. We see injuries where repetitive use causes the extremity to desynchronize and overheat ... to have a compensatory fulcrum ... to function in antagonism to the other side ... We give these situations a diverse number of fancy names ... often prescribing exercises that can only aggravate the health of the whole, because the whole is not synchronized and able to re-center and rebuild. We see shoulder damage in newborns. We see frozen shoulders that have lost all internal synchronization and freeze up like an engine with no oil. We see carpal tunnel syndromes ... et al. There is only one process that needs to be at work: the indwelling fluid dynamics that form the whole extremity ... Then we heal as wholeness is restored.

We will hopefully give you the tools and material to think and treat at a level rarely engaged in our profession. We will see familiar therapeutics and find the whole process quite simple and rewarding.

TREATMENT OF THE EXTREMITIES THROUGH THE MIDLINE

Section one: The Center and Peripheral Midlines

We all have received information on dermatomes and myotomes in our basic education. It is obvious that these segments relate to each other and find their position through some greater organizing intelligence. The intelligence is in itself a mystery, but we can realize through studying Sutherland, and our own experience, that the midline of the trunk and the midline in the extremities are connected at specific points. These points, or fulcrums, are the organizational lines of the blueprint of the Health.

Our evaluations will include this perfection, and also the compromised point of relationship from which the patient is actually functioning.

A working knowledge of the seventh cervical embryological segment and the limb buds is necessary, and worth your time and effort ...

TREATMENT OF THE EXTREMITIES AND PRIMARY RESPIRATION

Section Two: Power Points

This topic is new to the profession. Until Power Points were introduced, the extremities were treated using balanced ligamentous tension, without the support of the therapeutic forces of primary respiration ... balanced ligamentous tension was taught by Sutherland in his earlier years; he most likely received it from Dr. Still.

There are various forms of balanced ligamentous tension taught today. Some use barriers, some a variety of direct and indirect methods. Balanced ligamentous tension does not engage primary respiration. Anne Wales said that Will Sutherland did teach thoracic respiratory dynamics with the extremities; there was a direction in his work toward functional principles.

Later in his life, Sutherland began to incorporate his understanding of fluid dynamics, potency, and embryology into principles for treating the extremities. He called the process Power Points. I was introduced to Power Points by Ruby Day in 1984. Anne Wales later told me she had not learned this from Will because her husband was dying at the time (may he rest with her in eternity).

Apparently, the Sutherland Cranial Teaching Foundation was offered this information in 1990 and was not interested in it.

All we will teach you comes directly from Dr. Sutherland's study group. This group was composed of about fifteen people who were with him from 1935 until his death. These people traveled and taught with him. Only a few supported Magoun's teaching after Will died. Many, like Ruby Day, preferred the indirect approach and became silent after Will passed.

This study group was the core of Will's teaching legacy ... people like Alvera Miller, Alan Becker, Annie Biddle, Rollin Becker, George Laughlin, Anne Wales, Chester Handy, Harold Magoun, and Thomas Schooley were some of the names I was made familiar with.

Later, in 1990, I talked with Rollin, and he knew of the course of events that led to the development of the Power Points principles.

As you will notice, Sutherland draws heavily on the study of embryology in his discovery of these principles ... it is really as amazing as his other contributions. In this application, he introduces the midline into his work.

There are twelve comments that complete the picture of his work ... these are from Ruby, who got them from Will and made minor additions.

1. Know the bone ... this means the bone's history from conception to maturity. It includes figuring out the developmental axis (midline) of the bone that organizes the shape and tempo of growth.
2. Discern intraosseous motion in the bone. This is one of Sutherland's major insights. Motion inside the bone. Its metabolic breathing. He moves us away from the inertia, away from the compression into the Health, the breathing bone. The motion present inside the bone is a non-axial motion that occurs in three dimensions, not the biomechanical motion that Magoun presented.
3. Place the fingers with precision. The fingers need to meet the Power Point, which is the end of the internal midline around which the growth centers organize themselves. This precision is a key element. The index finger and the thumb form a "bird's beak," and the Power Point is inserted into the notch of the beak.

4. Tapping. This is a step I have added because the internal midline is not always easy to sense. What one can do is direct one's own Tide toward the center of the bone. The midline will react to the Tide and show itself, allowing one to align more precisely.
5. Sense the midline and align with it.
6. The midline floats like a cork on the sea.
7. Fluctuate the midline by moving the two ends in opposite directions.
8. A stillpoint will appear once the fluctuation brings itself to the fulcrum.
9. After the stillpoint, there will be automatic shifting inside the bone as the internal Zone B normalizes the metabolic fields of the bone, realigning the strain pattern.
10. The therapeutic forces appear to go outside the bone as the smaller Zone B and the larger fluid body merge.
11. After a pause, the bone will often correct the long axis dysfunctions. Sometimes it feels like the bone is yawning.
12. Return of normal intraosseous motion and a discernible shift in the lesion posture.

WGS NOTES FROM RUBY DAY

The following information was learned by Ruby Day from Dr. William Garner Sutherland from around 1935 to 1950. I received it while studying with her in 1984.

There are self-correcting forces and potency in the developmental axis (living midline) that are more important than the axis of motion.

Self-correcting forces will use different methods at different moments during a single treatment ... direct action, indirect action, opposing physiological motion, et cetera.

Attention is a vital function. We must concentrate, see the whole bone and the long axis. This opens a very large field of vision that expands beyond the local level to the whole.

Do not do somatic work after the Tide has done its work ... this will erase much of the treatment.

Dr. Sutherland was a kind, quiet man of few words.

Dr. Sutherland and Dr. Arbuckle dissolved their relationship ... WGS said conflict requires compassion. Foam is always blowing around on the surface of the ocean. The wind will dissipate it. The negativity in the world will be blown away by the wind until all of mankind is free and redeemed. The foam of conflict is always present in the world, just let the wind blow until the storm passes. Lesions are washed clean by the breath of the Tide.

Touch lightly.

The body knows more than we do. All we do is direct our attention in a precise manner.

The first course with WGS was two weeks ... one week of anatomy and one week for the CV4 ... the second year (1939) ... we had two weeks of technique and the vault hold ... year three he really gave it to us!

Read Alvera Miller and Charlotte Weaver.

Concerning Power Points ... he said, "The long axis in the bones is related to growth centers" ... the long axis is the field of balance ... therapeutic forces arise from this long axis midline ... the longitudinal forces are deep ... there is a vertical light correcting, balancing, and healing.

Being at two points on the axis creates a "gap" ... the gap is a visual impression which creates disengagement of both internal and external (inter articular) lesions. The bones swing themselves free. They do not move around the axis of motion (mechanical axis). We see the midline; it engages, fluctuates, and goes still ... at the stillpoint you must release your mind.

After the stillpoint, the bones change shape ... long then short ... breathing ... correcting ... rebalancing and healing ... remember, this replaces the mechanical axis!

Touch with attention; it has power.

The midline axis for the maxillary is in the frontal process.

The ethmoidal midline is in crista galli.

HIGHLIGHTS OF PHASE FIVE

Transformation of Consciousness

Fluid fields can lesion. –WGS

The head and upper neck develop as one region with several fluid segments.

Seams have different rates and carry the shape and power necessary to create and replenish functions.

Space is not empty.

Our awareness is a by-product of creation; our awareness must be transmuted.

Rebalancing – Zone B. The ocean and the shared stillness.

Automatic shifting is followed by emptiness, followed by the "light bulb going on."

Growth and development depend upon fluid fields acting freely.

Banana, can you feel it?

Can you feel cranial/pelvic biokinetics?

Eyes to the heart, then divide attention and observe breathing.

What is primary respiration?

PHASE SIX ... RELATED TOPICS

The Other Pair of Hands

Zone B evaluation: A to B, B without A, B with respirations, one drop, no distance, protoplasmic fluid body, body of fluids, health.

Levels of stillness: atmospheric, breathing 2–3 and fulcrum, dropping down into a deeper stillness ... the waiting room in the house under the sea ... the dynamic stillness, meeting with the presence as a healer, teacher (level four), see the mandala from Cathédrale de Fribourg ... stillpoints are beginnings ... then we meet the new landscape and we mature in our understanding.

Meditation: direction of easy thoracic respiration, balance point (neutral), ocean passing through suffusing thoracic respiration, after a while thoracic suffuses the ocean (the return of the soul to spirit), one embryonic breath.

Notation: our breathing is usually connected to worldly concerns and is not connected to our Health ... this exercise helps this, also attaching one's awareness to the voice behind the breathing.

The observers: perceptual studies.

Work without using any calories.

Protoplasm is dynamically still ... the Breath of Life suffuses it ... space opens in a form, function begins ... the wholeness of each diverse form appears and unfolds eternity in a lifetime.

Ignition is fire ... it brings life, form, and wisdom.

Vertex to xiphoid ... one egg-shaped fluid field.

Rebalancing: the fluid body and its fulcrum in the sea (from the feet).

Neutrals during extremity work usually relate to thoracic respiration.

Fulcrums are many things ... in a manner of speaking they are seeds ... in the seed is one, then, as it comes into being, there are sometimes two ... for example, one hand. The image is one hand but it appears in two places (i.e., two hands).

Rebuilding an extremity requires this:

- Fire ... ignition
- All function oriented to the midline ... tissue fluid and potency
- Capacity for neutral and automatic shifting

Think about involuntary consciousness:

- Space opens ... function moves in
- Stillpoints are beginnings ... they precede the incarnate process of eternity entering time ...
- We have two kinds of memory ... one in time and one in eternity

THE SEA AROUND US

In a dramatic message, Rachel Carson tells us a tremendously deep truth about nature and life. In her book *The Sea Around Us* (Oxford University Press, 1991), she almost passes the limits of our imagination when she speaks about molding liquid rocks fluctuating in a great tidal sea—a sea that has left its imprint in the hardened stones.

Who could imagine all the mountains of the earth as a liquid sea moved by a great Tide? The drama of heat, liquefaction, and transmutation goes beyond our imagination. And so it is with nature. She is wise and unpredictable. And so it is with the divine, an unimaginable mystery of love moving us always into the unexpected beyond our imaginations.

Osteopathy is like that. It seems like one settles into a comfortable belief system and is suddenly shaken from one's point of view. One is displaced into a deeper, richer understanding. One's whole life shifts. We are all on a ship at sea, with no known port of destination. Dr. Sutherland lived on the edge of an unknown sea.

In an effort to memorialize William Sutherland, I would like to reflect and comment upon the presence of Primary Respiration as a sea around us. My goal is to share my story in hopes it will validate others who have a deep sense of love for nature and God as the crucible in which we live. Man has boldly stepped away from his natural environment and polarized the divine into shameless dogma. In spite of our categorized beliefs, nature has a greater wisdom than man, especially a human race that manipulates its environment unsuccessfully.

The sea around us, and its infinite variety of motions and expressions, is our natural environment. Our awareness of it is a natural state of mind. Our immersion into it creates oneness.

Dr. Sutherland's wife created an oil painting for him. It reportedly depicted his understanding of the Tide. What I have been told is that this painting was a house under the sea with all the doors and windows open, and somewhere was assigned to it the words "My father's mansion has many rooms."

Since the mid-seventies the picture has inhabited my life as a riddle, as an inspiration, and as a fact. This image has made me comfortable when life has been too great to fathom, and finally this sea around us has become real for me.

The sea around us is more than a deep silence. Its presence is love. The story of how this happened I cannot say, because I cannot identify specific perceptual acts that brought it into focus for me. It came unexpectedly, yet it is always there. Even when unaware of it, one still knows the sea and its endlessness are present—the sea around us, our essential source of food, love, and becoming. This palpable living process creates a change in oneself unequaled by any form of healing. One simply becomes whole, transparent, and complete. One is awed by the intimate communion of life and its effect upon one's density, destiny, and capacity for change.

Osteopathy begins for us under our hands or between our hands. We learn to feel resistance and interface with it. We go to barriers, slowly, quickly, easily, and at times with frustration. If we are lucky, someone gives us a choice between barriers and direction of ease. If we persist, we learn that motion begets more motion, the whole moves the part, and the end point of treatment is not articular release but a change in the whole patient.

I began cranial work believing that Primary Respiration was inside the patient, when no one could agree upon where it was located. How one linked into it, other than through central nervous system–modulated activity, no one would say. One's only resolve was to go deeper. Little tribes emerged. Groups formed and argued about the bones, the fluid, and the potency; a hierarchy of frustration appeared and one felt obligated to seek out and explore these ideas. Why? Because the patients were responding.

The clinical results reflected a deeper truth. Bones, fluids, potency, layers in layers, always more precision. Motions—which one is therapeutic? Which wave is the wave? Converging themes, diverging applications. More physics, mysteries always hidden. Where is the fulcrum? We learn and learn, patients heal. We find ourselves faced with more difficult cases and an ego that feels threatened as it stops being the force behind the knowing and the action.

Those movements of truth then appear when the unexpected breaks into the treatment and shatters one's prior sense of what primary respiration is.

The unexpected movement of something outside of the patient, perhaps a silence, perhaps a distant fulcrum. One searches for answers. Certainly W. G. Sutherland and his students have left us hints that primary respiration is not inside the patient. Years pass between questions and the answer. One reference point during treatment shifts from inside to outside the patient. The outside presence of primary respiration enters our lives in moments other than during treatment. The validation of the presence of the sea around us follows us into the wilderness. It follows us into moments of being blessed by persons of pureheartedness, and slowly the sea merges into our hearts. Something outside of us begins to create our consciousness of the moment, and that created consciousness allows us to serve. One begins slowly to understand that consciousness is not a tool to be used, but an element of wisdom that is a mirror of the sea around us. One realizes one's consciousness has been transformed by the Tide and is held by the Tide and can be taken away by the Tide. In other words, our skill level lasts only while the Tide holds it, then the moment passes. The future is not guaranteed. In every treatment one begins as a beginner, and sometimes the sea is silent. Then its presence emerges. Sometimes there is an element of simplicity that makes the treatment brief.

Sometimes one enters into a stillpoint that seems to fill every point between oneself and the horizon. The moment lasts through the day and through the night. Even at night one feels this great sea around us all. Sometimes it recedes. Sometimes it ebbs with a silence as deep as forever. Sometimes it comes ashore swelling with presence and creating us, sustaining us. We are given a life of service.

I have never seen this painting of a house under the sea, but it has served to sustain me when my reason was fractured by reality. Hopefully my comments will help sustain the memory of a house under the sea with all the doors and windows open. This is the Tidal presence, the waters moving without a rate.

One pauses in the image of this painting. All the doors and windows are open and the great sea of love is passing through undiminished, but who opens the doors and the windows?

One pauses.

The answer lives in forever.

LAURENS VAN DER POST

"The answer must be sought first by the individual alone, as if it were in the desert of each of us. We have to accept this sense of something missing, however improbable or insignificant it may seem, as our guide towards distant life-giving waters."

The Heart of the Hunter, (1961)

"Human beings are perhaps never more frightening than when they are convinced beyond doubt that they are right."

The Lost World of the Kalahari,(1958)

"The spirit of man is nomad, his blood Bedouin, and love is the aboriginal tracker on the faded desert spoor of his lost self; and so I came to live my life not by conscious plan or prearranged design but as someone following the flight of a bird."

A Walk with a White Bushman, (1986)

PHASE SIX – THE OUTSIDE PRESENCE OF PRIMARY RESPIRATION, THE GENERATIVE FULCRUM, AND POWER POINTS

This Phase is a transitional period. We are moving from our own resources and ideas to those of primary respiration. We are becoming dependent upon the Tide. We have been inspired by many teachers to lean upon the Tide for the force and presence to create healing.

As we look back to Phase Four, we see it was there that we became aware that the Tide centers us. It gives us the awareness, patience, and love to participate in the drama of a treatment. This transition takes time and conceptual understanding.

We began in Phase Five to touch the void (dark emptiness). This is often disarming and confusing as one's consciousness relaxes into being still and knowing. This new knowing is empty of thoughts, motivation, or expectations, and our old mind will not shift easily. Why? Well, we have given control based upon our sense of necessity and as an adaptation to living in a materialistic world. We have also lost our true relationship with our Health (true self). As a result, we have ingrained in ourselves a sense of necessity that promotes being in control and not falling apart (i.e., going to neutral). Our work, therefore, is first to decide if we wish to be of service in this way or not. This is a transition of choice, not demand. One is free to find out that one is not free.

As we studied the midline, we realized that our consciousness must be transmuted by the Tide in order to see Zone D completely.

How often are you moved by the Tide? How has Zone D changed?

We are children of the Sea Around Us. The sea has a presence (a loving touch) that takes us well beyond the Long-Tide. We work with this in Phase Six. We also begin to study the movement of creation, as the sea creates the fulcrums from which function and form unfold. The interface between the fulcrum and the sea is a oneness of no distance. In this oneness there is a wholeness to the therapeutic process. We watch this happen.

We begin by reviewing the facial seams. We discover new truths as we follow this story of fluid body segmentation in places not noted in embryology texts, like the temporomandibular joint.

We observe thoracic respiration at different levels: the individual, the instinctual, the Health, and in communion with primary respiration. There is also a review of "centering around the edges," which helps us return to our original awareness of nature. This further exposes Zone D.

The sea is breathing us. The sea passes through us. It has a loving presence. We listen for this as it touches us.

PERCEPTUAL STATES CHART

PERCEPTUAL STATES

Intellect 8-14 CPM	Intuition 2-3 CPM	Instinct Long-Tide		Holy Stillness	Life
Mind is facilitated	Natural mind	Attention is moved by the long-tide; it breathes	TRANSMUTATION	heart awakens	The Incarnate Movement of Creation
Mind is full of thoughts, noisy, lesion orientated	Mind quiets easily but one is vulnerable to habits	Evolutionary mind		heart knows -- direction of ease	
Rational format, find lesion and resolve it	Intuitive skills evolve but vulnerable to emotions; intention is upon healing	Emotions replaced by Virtue, i.e., Compassion without Empathy		The Mystery becomes a snese of direction	
Emotionally unstable	Empathy is a challenge; fluid priority is clear	Instinctive awareness of Greater Mind with Intention to follow another will		soft peace	
Sensitivity fluctuates	Sensitivity presents but can be undisciplined	Sensitivity is extrasensorial and not limited by one's intention		sensory conversion	
Breathing is not synchronized with other rhythms ("thoracic" or forced abdominal); variable central nervous system motion	Breathing begins low ascends; quiet; brain quiets, centers	Thoracic respiration suffused by the Sea		two breaths die in a new breathing	
Observer is fixed on goal: intentions are fixed	Observer is less fixed, balanced but vulnerable to interpretation and labeling of patient's state	Observer holds still for short periods of time		Communion of mind	
Attention focal	Attention shifts with fluit; rapid eye movement possible	Beyond rapid eye movement; lucid consciousness		The dream emerges into reality through a veil	
Tune is paced by goals -- harried	Time is more fluid	Future comes like the wind		Forever still	
Memory is knowledge	Memory is more liquid but opaque			memory of Greatness	

SCHEMATIC OF THE FLUID FIELDS

Middle Face Fluid Field
Incus
Soft Palate
Alisphenoid
Maxilla
Zygoma
Temporal Bone
TMJ
McBride's Line
Infratentorial Fossa
Lower Tent
Cerebellum
Brainstem, Cranial Nerve Nuclei
Oral Pharnyx
Adenoids, Tonsils
Palatines, Teeth
Spinal Cord (C_{1-3})
Clavicle

Seam Between Middle and Lower Face Fluid Fields
Oral Cavity
Foregut
Sinuses
Lungs
Tongue
Foramen Magnum

Lower Face Fluid Field
Temporal Bone
T.M.J.
Malleolus
Mandible
Pouch – **Tongue (Invaginates,** Forms Thyroid)
Sphenomandibular ligament
C2C3

Muscles Moving Forward
Face, Tongue, Jaw, TMJ

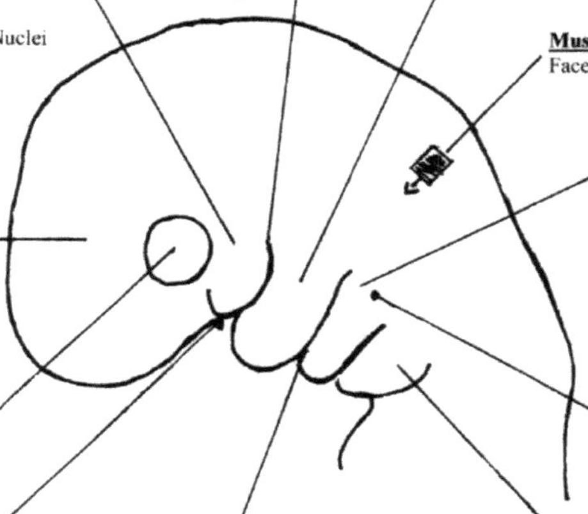

Upper Face Fluid Field
Supratentorial Space
Osseous, visceral
and neural tissue
TMJ
Upper Tent
Cerebrum
Sutherland Fulcrum
Anterior Tent
Temporal Bone

Hyoid Fluid Field
Ear
Stapes
Temporal Bone
Stylohyoid Ligament
Styloid Process, Jaw
Pouch – Tonsils
TMJ

Ear

Laryngeal Fluid Field et al
Mucosa Tongue
Posterior 1/3
Pouch – Thymus
Parathyroids
Hyoid
Pharynx
Larynx

Eye

Seam Between Lower Face & Hyoid Fluid Fields
Pinna of Ear
External Auditory Meatus
Pouch – Tympanic Cavity
Eustachian Tube

Seam Between Upper and Middle Face Fluid Fields
Invaginates – Nose, Philtriu **Philtrum**,
Frontal-Zygomatic Suture, Orbits
Eye
Temporomandibular Joint
Supratentorial-Infratentorial Interface
V3, Dreamer
Lamina Terminalis
Junction of Brainstem – Brain
Nasal Lacrimal Duct
Ethmoid Notch
Transverse Sinus

STRUCTURES PRESENTED HERE ARE NONANATOMICAL. THEY REFER TO THE FLUID FIELDS OF GROWTH AND DEVELOPMENT FOR THAT PARTICULAR FUNCTION.

MARK TWAIN'S SUPPORT FOR OSTEOPATHY

Around 1900, Mark Twain wrote in his notebook, "To ask a doctor's opinion of Osteopathy is equivalent to going to Satan for information about Christianity."

Twain developed an interest in Osteopathy after coming into contact with it in his hometown of Hannibal, Missouri. Dr. Still had an office in Hannibal for some months late in 1889, before setting up the American School of Osteopathy. In mid-1899 the Twain family took a trip to Europe. A little while before they left, Twain's second daughter, Jean Clemens, developed epilepsy. While they were in London, a friend urged Twain to seek the help of a Dr. Henrik Kellgren in Sweden. They continued on to Sweden, finally ending in Sennan, where Jean had treatment.

One pauses.

The answer lives in forever.

BIODYNAMICS OF OSTEOPATHY BOOK SERIES

This book is one of a series of twelve *Biodynamics of Osteopathy* books. It is recommended that you read the whole series in order, as each book builds on the understanding from prior books. It is also recommended that you seek experienced teachers and mentors to help you experience the full depth of the information given.

The full series is as follows:

Phase One is about involuntary motion, which is motion present in the whole and in the lesion. We learn to synchronize with the breathing of Primary Respiration before we approach any treatment. This synchronization is the key to working with stable rates and not irritating the system. The principle of synchronizing with a healthy aspect of the patient suffuses the whole teaching program. This synchronization shifts our awareness to a different level of receptivity, which allows us to see Primary Respiration rather than the lesion field, and this eventually leads us to an understanding of the intention of Primary Respiration.

Phase Two is about communication with the natural laws of healing that surround activity at 2 to 3 cycles per minute. We synchronize with the breathing of Primary Respiration and also add the skill of sensing the fulcrum, the Stillness through which the breathing creates form and function. It is a different kind of synchronization from that in Phase One, shifting our awareness more deeply. As this occurs, the treatment automatically expresses itself. The end point of treatment, when compared with Phase One, reveals several differences. We find this kind of synchronization works exclusively with the fluid body and the outcome of treatment is more complete than when working with tissue alone.

Phase Three is centered around the activities of the Long Tide (100 second cycle). We explore an indwelling therapeutic force already present in the lesion field. We learn that the dural system is not made-up of three sickles but rather a series of folds in a sac, arising during growth and development. We see the relationship between the upper and lower dural sacs, awakening us to the independence of two separate tentorium cerebelli. We discover that zone D, the horizon, and the Wire (along which the Long Tide moves during its intended therapeutic course) are all linked as natural laws pertaining to this level of Primary Respiration.

Phase Four focuses on the Midline, a place where the spatial relationships are expressed as a whole. It synchronizes and centers us in such a way that we become aware of Zone D and the Dynamic Stillness. The Third Level Stillness in Phase Four is different from the Stillness in the other Phases – we are centered by the Stillness at the center of creation. Our intention is replaced by the intention of the Tide which can facilitate our spiritual path.

Phase Five is about *the face*. As we approach the face, we use all of the principles that we have learned in Phase One, Two, Three, and Four. We work with automatic shifting and notice differences from how the face is viewed by older models within Osteopathy in the Cranial Field. As we synchronize with the therapeutic presence of the Long Tide we see what we can learn about the face from that landscape. We also work with Seams, Dynamic Stillness, and Ignition.

Phase Six is a continuation of our journey into the Wholeness that generates life and delivers therapeutic forces that transmute lesions once Neutral is expressed. It is a mixture of activities centered around the outside presence of Primary Respiration as something that is a non-biological force and that has a persona. We will also continue to explore seams and then move on to the extremities, first in the embryological terms and then as Sutherland taught them in his work called PowerPoints. Phase 6 is a time to build your understanding of the Tide and refine your skills.

Phase Seven highlights the Health. Dr. Still's famous comment "Find the Health; anyone can find disease," has plagued many minds over the last century. We come to the clear vision of several indwelling aspects of the Health: Love ... liquid light ... and a diamond matrix. A approach to the terminally ill and dying patient is addressed. In the somatic sensation of the Tide passing through the House Under the Sea, our awareness is transmuted by the Health. The lesion is seen as a precognitive act of the Health. Thoracic Respiration, Primary Respiration, and Ignition are as One. The landscape is vast ... and the principles of healing are even more substantial than we have previously experienced.

Phase Eight is a deeper exploration of seams, balanced rhythmic interchange, and the Flame of Intention as a therapeutic modality. Phase Eight is the culmination of our awareness of Wholeness, and ultimately brings us to the Divine Presence, Unconditional Love and Oneness. The living Tide dominates the awareness while forms move to the background. One feels the Breath of Creation in oneself as the Center of Wholeness. One feels the Unfoldment of oneself as one is Created. Our consciousness is a gift; we do not own it and if we try to control it we lose Wholeness.

Phase Nine is when we are able to fully evaluate and treat the Central Nervous System and the Eye. We also address Fire and the therapeutic modality of the Shakedown. True action is moved from Love and makes our perception exist. This Love is self-emptying and by its nature allows us to Serve as part of the Perfect. Perception can be used to Serve something other than ourselves. We have attempted to enter this balance point between the Perfect and the Disease ... it is a point where the whole of everything is suspended by Love as it works to incarnate the Complete. In the balance point of everything is The Intention of the Tide following the movement of the distortion back to a True relationship with the Blueprint of Life.

Pediatrics One explores how children grow as a whole, not in parts as we sometimes believe. Children live in the Direction of Ease of motion present in their fluid metabolic fields, otherwise they get uncomfortable and require assistance. Does your treatment directly support the whole, or does it assume to support the whole? We realize children are not adults and cannot be treated as adults are. We approach the therapeutic modality of the "Meeting Place", prenatal and postnatal periods, the treatment of the pelvis during pregnancy, fetal malposition and labor.

Pediatrics Two is where we deepen in the perceptive awareness necessary to approach the treatment of children. We deepen in our appreciation of Wholeness, the three levels of Stillness and the "Meeting Place". We approach "Desert Neutral", where therapeutics pass into the neutral substance, and a mystery unfolds as the breath of Divine love cascades as a therapeutic force across a night desert landscape, filling and leaving behind no visible effects. We further address treatment of the pelvis and the uterus during pregnancy. We explore thoracic and Primary Respiration in children, and the Family Circle.

Pediatrics Three is where we continue to study the therapeutic Flow of Attention. We deepen in Third Level Stillness and the Meeting Place. The Meeting Place is easily misinterpreted … our observer must be so still and neutral that the process can be seen as it happens. The central nervous system in the child can be finally approached for evaluation and treatment. We explore teething and also the "locked up head". We use the therapeutic modality of the Flame of Intention, and its connection to the Breath of Life. Everything is transparent to the Breath of Life.

ABOUT THE AUTHOR

James Jealous, D.O. (1943–2021), was an osteopathic physician, teacher, and writer. His life's work was founding and developing **Biodynamics of Osteopathy**, a unique methodology he established within the field of osteopathy, following the lineage of Dr. A.T. Still and Dr. W.G. Sutherland.

He was born in Saco, Maine, and since his father was an osteopathic physician, he was around osteopathy from an early age. He studied at Kirksville College of Osteopathic Medicine in Missouri (now the A.T. Still University of Health Sciences), graduating in 1970. He then set up practice in rural Maine as an osteopathic primary care physician.

Over time, Dr. Jealous saw parallels between the work of embryologist Dr. Erich Blechschmidt and that of osteopathic physician Dr. William Garner Sutherland. This inspiration led him to create his own body of work. In the early 1990s, he began teaching "A Biodynamic View of Osteopathy in the Cranial Field," which, as he developed his specific methodology, was refined to "Biodynamics of Osteopathy."

A deeply spiritual person, he felt most at home in the natural world and was an avid fisherman and hiker.

For more information, please visit:
https://BiodynamicsOfOsteopathy.com

There is a wind passing through ...
it is the motion of creation,
the eternal motion of Divine love.